# *The Dementia Caregiver's Survival Guide.*

*Unlock the Art of Caring With these Expert proven Strategies to soothe, Inspiring Coping Tips to conquer , and Everyday Practical Magic for a Fulfilling Adventure in Dementia Care.*

**Dr.Maria Martin**

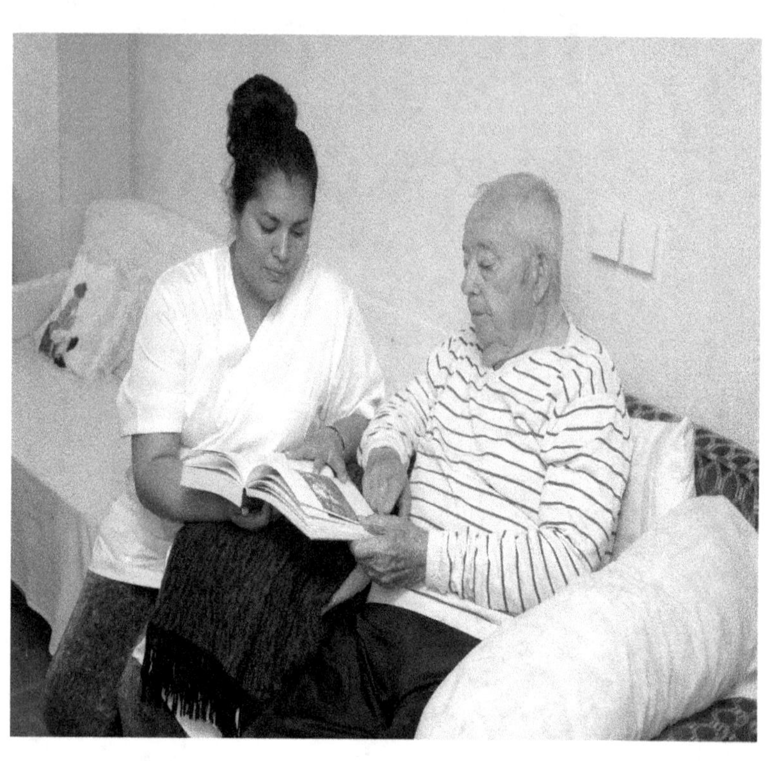

# Copyright [2024] [Dr.Maria Martin]

# Table of contents

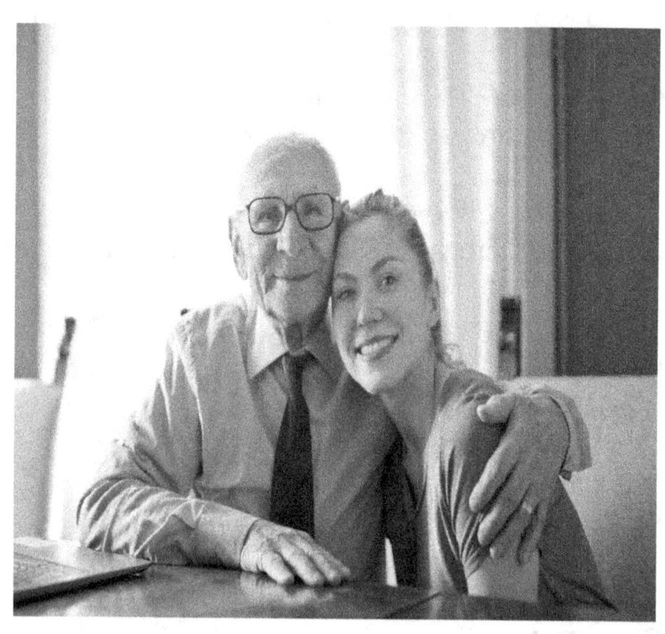

# *Introduction*

## *The Dementia Caregivers Survival Guide: Navigating the Path With Ease*

Dementia caring is a unique path fraught with difficulties and emotional complications. As we explore more into the complicated world of caring for people with dementia, it becomes clear that caregivers play an important role in offering support, affection, and help. This book provides a short but informative introduction of dementia caring, highlighting the critical necessity for a caregiver-specific survival guide.

# _Understanding of Dementia Caregiving_

Dementia, a disorder that affects memory, cognitive function, and everyday living, necessitates a tailored approach to caring. The obligations go well beyond just assisting with regular activities. Caregivers find themselves navigating a maze of emotions, from compassion to irritation, as they seek to offer the best care possible.

## _The heart of the matter: the need of a survival guide._

A survival guide serves as a compass for caregivers as they navigate the delicate dance of dementia caring. Why do we need such a guide? The significance stems from the many hurdles that caregivers endure on this one-of-a-kind journey.

### ▪ *Navigating the emotional roller coaster*

Caregivers often experience emotional upheaval. Their love for the person they are caring for is unshakable, but the everyday challenges may cause stress, worry, and even burnout. A survival guide acts as a lighthouse, providing coping techniques to deal with these emotional highs and lows.

### ▪ *Unravelling Dementia's Complexities*

Caregivers face an ever-changing environment as dementia progresses through different stages and forms. A survival guide serves as a road map, assisting caregivers in understanding the subtleties of each stage and recommending specific solutions for successful caring.

### ▪ *The Silent Toll on Caregiver Well Being*

Caregivers often disregard their own health while caring for a loved one. Self-care is essential and cannot be stressed. A survival guide not only recognizes this, but also gives caregivers practical advice and encouragement to prioritise their mental and physical health.

- *Establishing a Support Network*

Caregivers often experience feelings of isolation. Being alone on this path might be intimidating. A survival guide advises caregivers to form a support system by interacting with people who understand the particular difficulties of dementia care.

- *Compassionate Approach*

A survival guide's value stems not only from its practical counsel, but also from its caring attitude. Caregivers are not alone in their problems, and a well-written handbook transmits this message sympathetically.

- *Educating and empowering caregivers*

Knowledge is an extremely strong instrument. A survival guide provides caregivers with the information they need to offer the best care possible. The book provides caregivers with the knowledge they need to succeed, from recognizing the complexities of dementia to developing successful communication methods.

- *Enhancing Resilience*

Caregiving is a marathon rather than a sprint. This lengthy voyage will need resilience. A survival guide builds resilience by creating confidence, providing solutions for overcoming hurdles, and emphasising the minor successes that make the caring experience worthwhile.

- *A Guide for Caregivers.*

Finally, the dementia caregiver's survival guide is more than simply a guidebook; it serves as a guiding beacon. It illuminates the way for caregivers, offering insights, techniques, and support. As we delve into the complexities of dementia caring in this book, keep in mind that the guide is more than simply a tool; it is a companion, travelling beside caregivers on their noble and arduous quest.

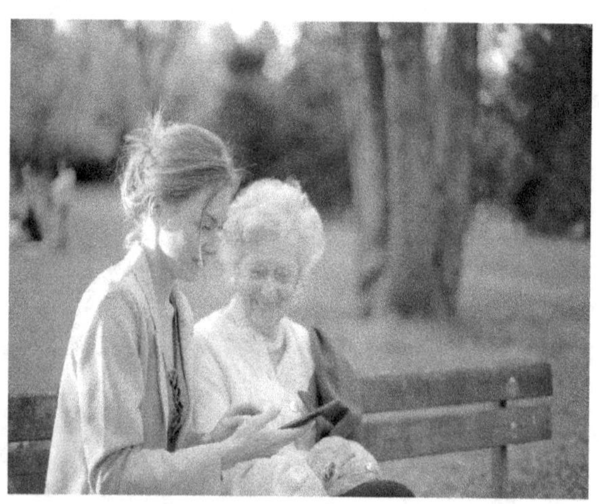

# Chapter 1

# Understanding Dementia: A Complete Exploration of Types, Stages, and Impact

Dementia is a complicated and diverse disorder that has a significant impact on both persons and their caregivers. In this chapter of dementia, we will look at the complexities of what dementia is, how it affects people, and the numerous forms and phases that define this difficult illness.

## Defining dementia

Dementia is not a single illness, but rather an umbrella term encompassing a variety of cognitive deficits that interfere with everyday activities. It is distinguished by a deterioration in memory, cognitive function, and capacity to accomplish daily tasks. Dementia is increasingly frequent in older persons, although it is not a natural aspect of ageing.

- *The Impact on Individuals*

Dementia has a major influence on people's life, influencing many facets of it. Memory loss, communication difficulties, and problems with problem solving are common consequences of cognitive decline. As the illness worsens, people may suffer personality changes, mood fluctuations, and a deterioration in their ability to manage their everyday lives.

- *Emotional and Psychological Impact*

Dementia not only impairs cognitive skills but also has an emotional impact on persons. The frustration of not being able to recall, the dread of the unknown, and the loss of independence may all contribute to anxiety, melancholy, and feelings of loneliness.

- ***Stress on Relationships***

Relationships between dementia patients and their loved ones may be strained. Communication becomes difficult, and roles within the family may change. Family members and caregivers bear a heavy emotional load as they observe their loved one's deterioration.

## *Different Types of Dementia*

Dementia is not one-size-fits-all. There are many varieties, each with its own unique traits and underlying reasons. Understanding these categories is critical for providing treatment and assistance to each individual's unique requirements.

- *Alzheimer's disease*

Alzheimer's disease is the most prevalent kind of dementia, accounting for 60–80% of cases. The formation of plaques and tangles in the brain causes nerve cell loss. Memory loss and cognitive deterioration are significant aspects of Alzheimer's disease.

- *Vascular dementia*

Vascular dementia is caused by impaired blood supply to the brain, which is often the consequence of strokes or other vascular disorders. The symptoms vary depending on which part of the brain is injured, but they may include issues with thinking, planning, and remembering.

- *Lewy Body Dementia.*

Lewy body dementia is defined by the presence of aberrant protein deposits in the brain known as Lewy bodies. Individuals with this kind of dementia may have hallucinations, motor problems, and shifts in awareness and concentration.

**▪ Frontotemporal dementia.**

Frontotemporal dementia is predominantly affecting the frontal and temporal lobes of the brain. It causes changes in personality, conduct, and linguistic abilities. Unlike Alzheimer's, it usually develops at a younger age, between 40 and 65.

**▪ *Mixed dementia.***

Mixed dementia is a mix of multiple forms, most often Alzheimer's disease and vascular dementia. The presence of overlapping symptoms complicates diagnosis and treatment.

## *Stages of Dementia*

Dementia progresses through many phases based on the severity of symptoms and their influence on everyday living. Understanding these phases allows caregivers to anticipate issues and offer appropriate assistance.

- *Early stage*

Individuals may continue to operate independently in the early stages, although modest cognitive alterations emerge. They may have difficulties recalling names or finding the appropriate phrases. Loved ones may detect changes in mood or conduct.

- *Middle Stage.*

As dementia develops to the middle stage, people need greater help with everyday duties. Memory loss worsens, and people may fail to recognize familiar persons or locations.

Behavioural signs such as wandering and irritability may develop.

- ***Late stage.***

The late stage of dementia is distinguished by substantial cognitive deterioration and a dramatic effect on everyday functioning. Individuals may lose their verbal communication skills, need help with all daily tasks, and endure physical deterioration.

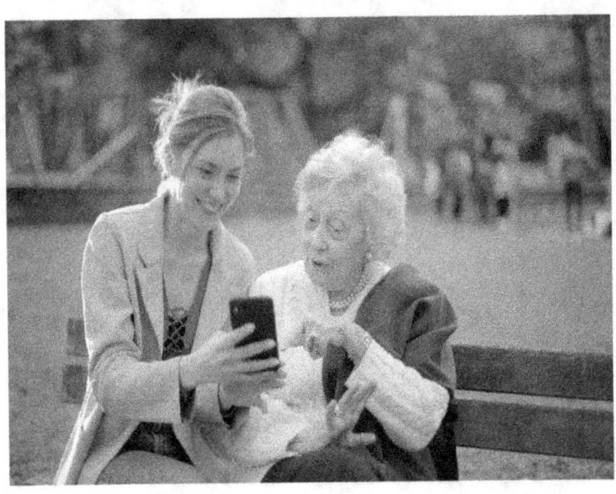

# *Chapter 2*

# *The Unsung Heroes: Understanding the Role of a Dementia Caregivers*

Caring for someone with dementia is a complex and difficult duty that demands unrivalled devotion and compassion. In this section, we will look at the enormous obligations and problems that dementia caregivers confront, as well as the mental and physical toll that comes with this noble but difficult journey.

## *Responsibilities of Dementia Caregivers:*

Dementia caring involves a wide range of tasks that go beyond standard caregiver obligations. It requires a distinct set of talents, empathy, and an unshakable dedication to improving the quality of life for people with dementia. Let's look at the key tasks that characterise the position of a dementia caregiver.

- *Help with daily tasks.*

Dementia often impairs a person's capacity to conduct ordinary tasks independently. Caregivers come in to help with bathing, clothing, grooming, and food preparation. Creating a secure and pleasant atmosphere becomes a primary focus.

- *Medication management*

Many people with dementia use medication to control symptoms and delay the course of the disease. Caregivers are responsible for arranging, administering, and monitoring drugs, ensuring that the person follows recommended regimens.

- *Emotional support*

As cognitive functions deteriorate, persons with dementia may feel increased emotions, disorientation, and irritation. Caregivers serve as an emotional anchor, bringing comfort, reassurance, and understanding in times of difficulty.

- *Facilitated Communication*

Effective communication gets more difficult as dementia advances. Caregivers use patience and creativity to promote communication by using gestures, visual aids, and a soothing tone to connect with the person.

- *Supervision and Safety*

Due to the potential of straying and safety issues, continual monitoring is typically required. Caregivers make sure the environment is safe, put in place safety precautions, and stay alert to avoid accidents or injuries.

- *Engaging in Meaningful Activities.*

Individuals with dementia need cognitive stimulation to function properly. Caregivers create and execute activities that are tailored to the individual's interests, creating engagement and a feeling of purpose.

- *Coordinating Healthcare Services.*

Caregivers serve as liaisons between individuals with dementia and healthcare providers. They make appointments, provide important information, and advocate for the best possible treatment.

- *Advocacy for Quality Of Life*

Caregivers advocate for the individual's overall health and quality of life. This involves meeting social, emotional, and recreational requirements in order to live a meaningful and enriching life.

## *Challenges for Caregivers of Dementia Patients*

The work of a dementia caregiver is not without its difficulties, and managing the complexity of caring may have an impact on both the caregiver's physical and emotional well-being.

### ▪ *Emotional Strain*

Witnessing a loved one's cognitive decline and personality changes may be emotionally taxing. Caregivers may experience loss, frustration, and helplessness as they adjust to the changing requirements of the dementia patient.

### ▪ *Physical Exhaustion*

The physical demands of caring, such as lifting, assistance with movement, and managing everyday duties, may contribute to fatigue. Caregivers often have to strike a balance between these expectations and their own needs for relaxation and self-care.

- *Financial stress.*

Providing care for someone with dementia may incur extra costs, such as medical bills, home renovations, and professional help. Caregivers may experience financial stress as they handle their new financial duties.

- *Social isolation*

Caregivers may experience social isolation due to the obligations of caring. Caregivers may feel isolated from friends and family as they struggle to balance their caring obligations with personal connections.

- *A lack of resources and support*

Accessing the right resources and support services is critical for successful caring. Unfortunately, caregivers may have difficulty getting enough support, resulting in emotions of frustration and stress.

- *Impact on Career and Personal Life.*

Balancing caregiving responsibilities with professional obligations and personal life is a tricky act. Many caregivers make compromises in both their professional and personal lives, resulting in job setbacks and relationship tensions.

## *The emotional and physical toll on caregivers*

- *Emotional impact*

- ***Guilt and grief:*** Caregivers may feel guilty about their inability to do more or about the feelings they are experiencing, such as annoyance or impatience. Furthermore, as dementia develops, caregivers may mourn the loss of someone they once knew.

- ***Burnout and Compassion fatigue:*** The constant demands of caring may result in burnout, which is characterised by physical and mental tiredness. Compassion fatigue, a kind of burnout related to caring, may sap a caregiver's empathy and resilience.

- *Physical Impact*
  - Lack of sleep: Caregivers may suffer from chronic sleep deprivation due to the irregular sleep patterns and nightly interruptions that are frequent in

dementia care. This increases physical weariness and exacerbates the emotional toll.

- *Health Compromise*

Caregivers often face the issue of neglecting their own health. Stress and tiredness may weaken the caregiver's immune system, making them more prone to sickness.

- *Effects on Relationships*

Caregiving obligations may strain relationships with friends, family, and even the individual being cared for. Caregivers may feel alone and struggle to strike a balance between caring tasks and social interactions.

# *Coping Strategies and Self-Care for Caregivers with Dementia*

Recognizing the difficulties experienced by dementia caregivers, it is critical to investigate coping mechanisms and emphasise the significance of self-care in order to reduce the mental and physical toll.

- *Create a Support Network*

Creating a support network of friends, family, and caregivers allows you to share your experiences while also gaining understanding and empathy.

- *Seek professional help.*

Engaging healthcare experts, counsellors, or support groups may provide useful direction and emotional support, recognizing the complexities of the caregiver's position.

- *Create realistic expectations.*

Understanding the limits of caring and creating reasonable goals for oneself is critical. Acceptance of the circumstance empowers caregivers to face obstacles with more resilience.

- *Prioritise Self-Care.*

Caregivers must emphasise self-care to preserve their physical and mental well. This involves obtaining enough sleep, participating in recreational activities, and seeking out moments of calm.

- *Discover Respite Care Options*

Respite care enables caregivers to take breaks while ensuring that the person with dementia gets excellent care. This short break is critical for avoiding burnout.

# Chapter 3

# "Mastering the Art of Caregiving: Expert Strategies for Effective and Sustainable Support"

Caring for someone with dementia is a complex and demanding duty that frequently demands more than good intentions. In this section, we will dig into the world of expert caregiving tactics, unravelling the professional guidance that supports good care and the critical function of developing a strong support network for both caregivers and people they care for.

# *Professional Advice for Effective Caregiving*

Caring for someone with dementia requires a skill set that extends beyond basic caring techniques. Expert plans, developed by the views of healthcare professionals and experts, are critical to delivering excellent treatment. Let's look at the main expert guidance that underpins good caring.

- *Understanding the individual's unique needs*
Every person with dementia is unique, and recognizing their special requirements is critical. Healthcare practitioners highlight the significance of personalising treatment to each person's preferences, habits, and history. A tailored approach guarantees that caring treatments are both successful and respectful of the person's dignity.

- *Effective Communication Skills*

Communication gets more difficult as dementia advances. Expert guidance often focuses on using clear and succinct language, keeping a calm tone, and using nonverbal clues to improve comprehension. These tactics promote meaningful interactions while reducing irritation for both caregiver and person.

- *Establishing A Structured Routine*

Establishing a defined schedule gives people with dementia a feeling of predictability and stability. Professionals suggest making a daily routine that includes regular meal times, activities, and rest intervals. Routine consistency is beneficial in reducing confusion and anxiety.

- *Fostering Independence within Limits*

While dementia may impair certain capacities, it is critical to promote independence whenever feasible. Expert solutions include striking a balance between assisting the person and letting them participate in activities that enhance their feeling of self-worth.

- *Managing Difficult Behaviours*

Dementia may cause problematic behaviours like hostility or irritability. Professionals urge caregivers to identify triggers, maintain patience, and use redirection tactics. Understanding the underlying reasons of problematic behaviours is critical for creating successful management methods.

- *Creating A Positive and Supportive Environment*

Individuals with dementia benefit greatly from a cheerful and supportive atmosphere. Experts recommend introducing things that elicit familiar and soothing feelings, such as beloved music, images, or fragrances. A well-designed setting fosters a feeling of safety and belonging.

■ *Utilising Technological Aids*

Advancements in technology provide significant tools for dementia care. Professionals propose adopting apps, reminder systems, and monitoring gadgets to improve safety and make care easier. Technological assistance may augment and enhance caring efforts.

■ *Regular Check-ins with Healthcare Professionals.*

Maintaining open channels of contact with healthcare experts is essential. Regular check-ins enable caregivers to get advice, review changes in the individual's health, and address any issues or problems they may be encountering. Collaboration with healthcare professionals promotes a comprehensive approach to care.

## *Developing a Support Network*

Caregiving is not a solo endeavour, but rather a communal one that benefits from the strength of a support network. Building and sustaining this network is critical for the well-being of both the caregiver and the dementia patient. Let's look at the components of developing a strong support network.

- *Family and Friends as Allies.*

Family and friends are an important part of the caregiver's support system. Open communication and enlisting loved ones in caring promote a feeling of shared responsibility. Emotional and practical assistance from family and friends may help reduce the stresses of caring.

## Caregivers' Support Groups

Participating in caregiver support groups allows others who face similar issues to share their experiences, ideas, and coping skills. These organisations provide a secure environment for emotional expression while also encouraging a feeling of belonging and understanding.

- ### *Professional support services.*

Engaging professional support services, such as home health aides or respite care, gives caregivers much-needed breaks and help. These programs benefit both the caregiver and the client with dementia.

- ### *Educational Resources*

Access to educational materials about dementia and caring is empowering. Workshops, seminars, and online courses provide useful insights into current caring approaches and research results. Continuous learning prepares caregivers to adapt to the individual's changing demands.

### ■ *Making Good Use of Community Resources*

Communities often provide tools particularly targeted for dementia caregivers. Adult day care programs, transportation services, and local dementia support groups are all possible options. Leveraging these resources improves the caregiver's capacity to deliver complete care.

### ■ *Financial and Legal Advisors*

Navigating the financial and legal elements of caring may be difficult. Seeking counsel from financial and legal specialists enables caregivers to make educated choices and prepare for their future. Addressing these issues results in a more secure caring journey.

**▪ *Counseling and mental health support***

Caregivers may encounter emotional difficulties, stress, and fatigue. Seeking therapy or mental health help is not a sign of weakness, but rather an active move toward emotional well-being. Professional counselling services provide caregivers a safe area to vent their emotions and get advice.

**▪ *Encouraging community participation***

It is good to encourage both caregivers and dementia patients to participate in the community. Participating in community events, religious activities, or social meetings fosters a feeling of belonging while combating social isolation.

# Chapter 4

# The Art of Serenity: Exploring Relaxation Techniques in Dementia Care

Caring for people with dementia requires a thorough awareness of the effectiveness of calming strategies. In this chapter , we will look at the value of soothing activities for both caregivers and dementia patients. We will also discuss the significance of providing a tranquil atmosphere and the transforming effect it may have on the well-being of persons navigating the difficult terrain of dementia.

# *Calming activities for caregivers and individuals with dementia*

- ***Engaging in Gentle Physical Activity***

Physical exercises may be quite relaxing for both caregivers and dementia patients. Simple activities such as simple stretches, tai chi, or brief walks may help you relax, boost your mood, and feel better overall.

- ***Musical Therapy***

The healing influence of music is well understood. Caregivers may include relaxing music into their daily routine, tailoring it to the individual's preferences. Calming melodies have the power to elicit happy feelings, relieve tension, and foster a peaceful environment.

- ***Aromatherapy***

The sense of smell is an extremely potent instrument for evoking memories and emotions.

Aromatherapy makes use of smells such as lavender or chamomile, which are recognized for their relaxing effects. Caregivers might use essential oils or scented candles to provide a comforting olfactory experience.

- *Meditation and Relaxation Techniques*

Introducing mindfulness and relaxation practices into the daily routine helps both the caregiver and the dementia patient. Deep breathing, meditation, and guided visualisation are all practices that enhance relaxation and reduce stress.

- *Art and craft activities.*

Drawing, painting, and creating are all creative pursuits that may be soothing. These activities allow for self-expression, boost cognitive function, and create a feeling of achievement, all of which contribute to a peaceful atmosphere.

- *Outdoor Activities*

Bringing the outdoors in or taking a leisurely walk around a garden may be really relaxing. Nature-based hobbies, such as bird watching or indoor plant care, provide a link to the natural world and promote relaxation.

- *Pleasant Sensory Experiences*

The sense of warmth may be quite relaxing. To promote physical comfort, caregivers might use warm blankets, heating pads, or comfy socks. Warmth not only soothes the body but also install a feeling of safety.

- *Using Pet Therapy*

Interactions with animals, often known as pet therapy, have shown to be quite beneficial in dementia care. Animals, whether they be a therapy dog or a gentle cat, may provide pleasure, friendship, and a sense of serenity.

- *Basic Massage and Touch*

Gentle contact, such as hand massages or shoulder rubs, may be very calming. Human contact fosters emotions of connection, decreases anxiety, and improves emotional well-being for both caregivers and dementia patients.

## *The Value of Creating a Peaceful Environment*

- *Reduced Stimuli*

Dementia patients may get overwhelmed by overwhelming stimulation. Creating a calm atmosphere entails limiting noise, decreasing clutter, and maintaining a well-organised place. A tranquil environment improves attention, decreases stress, and promotes general well-being.

- *Soft light*

Individuals with dementia may find harsh illumination disturbing. Soft, natural lighting helps to create a relaxing ambiance. Caregivers may utilise curtains, shades, or soft lighting to create a soothing atmosphere.

*Comfortable and familiar environments.*

It is critical to design environments that are both comfortable and familiar. Familiar things, treasured possessions, and individualised design provide a feeling of continuity, minimising confusion and fostering tranquillity.

- *Maintaining Consistent Routines*

Individuals with dementia benefit from having regular routines in place. Predictability in daily activities, mealtimes, and rest intervals fosters a feeling of security, lowering worry and fostering tranquillity.

- *Increasing Quiet Time*

In a world full of continual stimuli, making time for stillness is crucial. Caregivers may set aside times for peaceful activities, enabling both the caregiver and the dementia patient to rest and find consolation.

- *Sensory Stations That Are Personalized*

Creating bespoke sensory stations based on the individual's preferences is an effective soothing technique. These stations might contain things with different textures, relaxing smells, or familiar objects that bring back good memories.

- *Comfortable Furniture and Bedding*

Making sure the furniture is comfy and the bedding is attractive helps to create a serene atmosphere. Well-chosen furniture gives physical comfort, while a comfortable bed encourages peaceful sleep, which is necessary for emotional well-being.

■ *Increasing safety and security.*

A calm atmosphere is one that values safety and security. This includes reducing fall risks, guarding possible dangers, and making the person feel safe and cared for.

■ *Promoting a Positive Environment*

The entire mood of the caregiving setting is important for creating tranquillity. Caregivers may instil optimism by using encouraging words, uplifting décor, and maintaining a patient and understanding attitude.

## *Incorporating Relaxation Techniques into Daily Care*

■ *Observation and adaptability*

Observation is essential in determining which calming approaches are most effective for each person. Caregivers should monitor responses, preferences, and mood changes and modify calming activities appropriately.

### ▪ *Communication with healthcare professionals*

Communication with healthcare experts is vital. Caregivers might seek advice on how to customise calming tactics to the individual's unique requirements while ensuring that the strategies are consistent with overall care goals.

### ▪ *Collaboration With the Support Network*

Incorporating calming approaches into everyday care necessitates coordination with the support system. Family members, friends, and professional caregivers may all offer ideas and efforts to help create a relaxing and supportive atmosphere.

- *Approachable Flexibility*

Individuals suffering from dementia may react differently to various calming approaches at different periods. Caregivers should be adaptable in their approach, willing to test new tactics and alter them in response to the individual's changing requirements.

- *Recognizing little victories*

Small accomplishments are celebrated along the way to implementing relaxing practices. Celebrating these victories, whether they be a moment of quiet or a favourable reaction to a specific activity, promotes the efficacy of the selected tactics.

# Chapter 5

# Navigating the Storm: Inspiring Coping Tips for Dementia Caregivers.

Caring for someone with dementia presents several obstacles and emotional complications. In this chapter, we will look at inspirational coping methods for dementia caregivers, with an emphasis on coping mechanisms for dealing with stress and emotional issues. The significance of having a positive mentality will be highlighted, giving caregivers useful insights on building resilience and finding inspiration in the midst of a storm.

## Coping Mechanisms to Deal with Stress and Emotional Challenges

- *Mindful Breathing and Relaxation Methods*

In times of high stress, adopting mindful breathing and relaxation practices may be life-changing. Taking calm, deep breaths and concentrating on the present moment may help caregivers restore their composure and negotiate emotional issues with more clarity.

- *Establishing realistic expectations.*

Setting reasonable expectations is an essential component of good coping. Caregivers often feel pressured to do it all, but accepting limits and setting reasonable objectives reduces stress and develops a feeling of success.

- *Seeking social support.*

Caregivers often struggle with isolation. Building and maintaining a solid support network of family, friends, and other caregivers is an important outlet for sharing experiences, asking advice, and getting emotional support during difficult times.

- ***Engaging in Regular Physical Exercise.***

Physical activity is an effective stress reducer. Caregivers may add regular exercise into their routine, whether it's a brisk stroll, yoga, or another kind of physical activity they love. Exercise not only improves physical health but also boosts mood and mental well-being.

- ***Prioritising Self-Care***

Caregivers cannot afford to neglect their own needs. Taking time for oneself, whether by reading a book, engaging in a hobby, or just relaxing, is critical for emotional resiliency. Neglecting self-care may result in burnout, stressing the significance of prioritising personal well-being.

■ *Expressing Emotions via Creative Outlets*

Creativity is a wonderful way to handle emotions. Caregivers may express their emotions via creative hobbies like writing, painting, or music, which provides a cathartic release and promotes emotional well-being.

■ *Attending Support Groups and Workshops.*

Participating in support groups and programs designed for dementia caregivers fosters a feeling of community. Sharing experiences, learning from others, and receiving insights from specialists all add to a sense of understanding and validation while also providing coping techniques and tactics.

■ *Setting Boundaries and Asking for Assistance*

Recognizing the value of establishing limits is critical for caregiver well-being. Knowing when to ask for assistance and distribute chores helps parents avoid feelings of overload and handle their jobs with more balance and resilience.

## Maintaining A Positive Mindset

- ### Focusing on Small Victories

Celebrating minor accomplishments provides a source of encouragement for dementia caregivers. Recognizing and appreciating pleasant events, no matter how tiny, helps to keep an optimistic mindset in the face of adversity.

- ### Practising gratitude

Developing a feeling of appreciation is a transforming coping method. Caregivers might maintain a gratitude notebook in which they reflect on times of pleasure, compassion, and personal strengths. This practice encourages positivity and resilience.

- *Accepting Flexibility and Adaptability*.

Flexibility is an essential component of maintaining a positive attitude. Dementia caregiving is unpredictable, and adapting to changing circumstances with grace and resilience enables caregivers to approach challenges more optimistically.

- *Focusing on the Present Moment*

Dwelling on future uncertainties or past challenges can increase stress. Maintaining a positive mindset entails focusing on the present moment, appreciating the here and now, and finding joy in the immediate experiences of caregiving.

- *Developing A Sense of Humor*

Humour is a very effective coping mechanism. Finding moments of levity in the midst of difficulties reduces the emotional load and adds joy to caring. Humour, whether shared jokes, funny stories, or lighthearted activities, can be uplifting.

- ***Increasing Resilience through Reflection***

Reflecting on personal development and resilience is a source of inspiration. Caregivers can reflect on their journey, acknowledge their progress, and recognize the strength and adaptability that emerged as a result of the challenges.

- ***Cherishing Moments of Connection***

Connection to the person being cared for is a powerful motivator. Focusing on moments of connection, shared laughter, or meaningful interactions reinforces the benefits of caregiving and improves the caregiver's emotional well-being.

**▪ *Ensuring a Healthy Work-Life Balance***

Balancing caregiving responsibilities with personal life is essential for maintaining a positive attitude. Caregivers should strive for a healthy work-life balance by making time for personal interests, relationships, and activities that bring them joy and fulfilment.

## *Integrating Coping Tips Into Daily Care*

**▪ *Consistent Self-Reflection***

Regular self-reflection enables caregivers to assess their emotional well-being and identify areas where they may require additional assistance. Taking time for introspection increases self-awareness and guides the integration of coping strategies into daily life.

### *Open communication with the support network.*

Effective communication with the support network is critical. Caregivers should discuss their coping needs and preferences with family, friends, and professionals in order to foster a collaborative and understanding approach to emotional well-being.

### *Coping Strategies: Adaptability and Flexibility*

Coping strategies are not universally applicable. Caregivers should be willing to adapt and evolve their coping strategies in response to the changing needs of the individual with dementia as well as their own changing circumstances.

- *Schedule regular check-ins with healthcare professionals*

Regular check-ins with healthcare professionals ensure that coping strategies are consistent with overall care plans. Professionals can offer personalised advice, stress management tips, and additional resources to improve emotional well-being.

- *Celebrating Personal Development and Resilience*

Recognizing personal growth and resilience should be an ongoing process. Caregivers can keep a journal or reflection space to commemorate milestones, coping successes, and moments of inspiration that occur throughout their caregiving journey.

As caregivers embark on the difficult but rewarding journey of dementia caregiving, these uplifting coping strategies serve as beacons of strength. Fostering emotional well-being and maintaining a positive mindset are not only good for the caregiver's health, but they also help to create a nurturing and uplifting environment for the person with dementia.

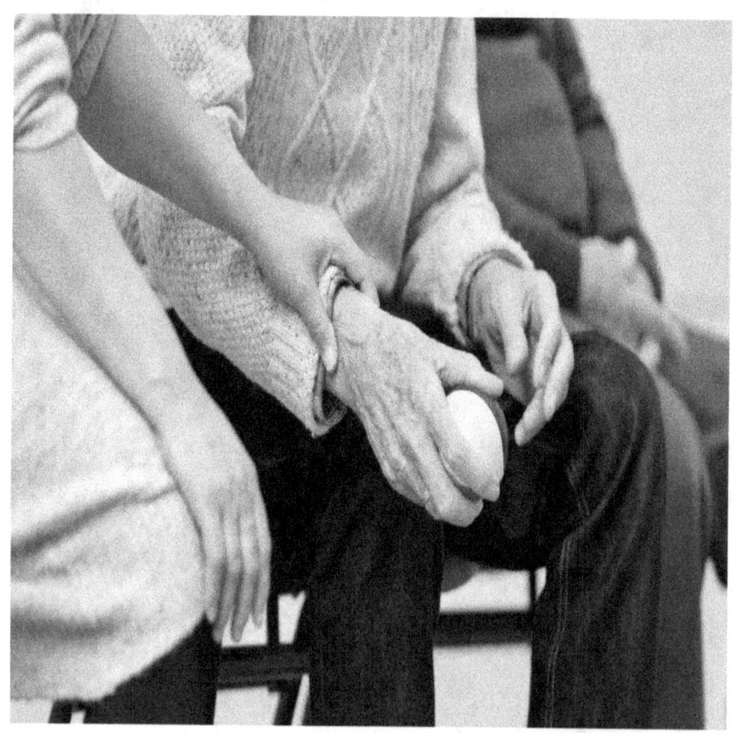

# Chapter 6

# *Practical Magic: Expert Tips for Managing Dementia on a Daily Basis*

Caring for people with dementia necessitates a unique combination of compassion, resilience, and a touch of practical magic. In this exploration, we will look at practical tips and tricks for dementia caregiving. These strategies are intended to make the caregiving journey more manageable by teaching caregivers how to provide effective and compassionate care while navigating the complexities of dementia.

# *Practical Tips for Daily Dementia Care:*

- ***Establish Consistent Routines***

Consistency is a critical component of effective dementia care. Establishing daily routines gives dementia patients a sense of predictability and security. Caregivers should create meal, activity, and rest schedules to reduce confusion and promote a structured environment.

- ***Producing visual and auditory cues***

Visual and auditory cues improve communication and understanding. Simple cues, such as labelling drawers or using colour-coded objects, aid dementia patients in navigating their surroundings. Auditory cues, such as gentle reminders or familiar sounds, can boost awareness and engagement.

■ *Simplified Communication Strategies.*

As dementia progresses, communication becomes increasingly difficult. Caregivers should use simplified communication strategies, such as clear and concise language, avoiding complex sentences, and incorporating gestures and facial expressions to convey meaning.

■ *Effective medication management*

Managing medications is an essential part of dementia care. Caregivers should create a medication management system that includes tools such as pill organisers and reminders. Regular communication with healthcare professionals helps to ensure that prescribed regimens are followed.

■ *Providing a Safe Living Environment*

In dementia care, safety is the most important consideration. Caregivers should inspect the living environment for potential hazards, install safety features such as handrails and non slip mats, and consider making home modifications to create a safe and supportive environment.

- ***Promoting Independence Within Limits***

While dementia may impair some abilities, caregivers should promote independence whenever possible. Simple modifications, such as providing easy-to-use utensils or incorporating visual prompts, allow people with dementia to participate in daily activities more independently.

### *Promoting Nutritional and Hydration Habits*

Maintaining good nutrition and hydration is critical for overall health. Caregivers should provide nutritious meals, ensure adequate fluid intake, and monitor dietary needs. Creative approaches, such as visually appealing presentations, can improve the dining experience.

### ▪ *Conducting Purposeful and Meaningful Activities*

Engaging individuals with dementia in purposeful activities improves cognitive stimulation and fosters a sense of accomplishment. Caregivers should tailor activities to the person's interests, including hobbies, music, and familiar routines.

### ▪ *Using Assistive Technology*

Advances in assistive technologies provide useful tools for dementia care. Caregivers can look into apps, devices, and sensors that improve safety, monitor health metrics, and provide cognitive stimulation.

### ▪ *Establishing a Comfortable Sleep Environment*

Quality sleep is critical for cognitive function and emotional well-being. Caregivers should establish a calming bedtime routine, create a comfortable sleep environment, and consult with healthcare professionals if they experience insomnia or nighttime disturbances.

## *Making the Caregiving Journey more manageable*

- *Creating realistic expectations.*

The journey of dementia caregiving presents unique challenges. Setting realistic expectations is essential. Caregivers should recognize their own limitations, seek assistance when necessary, and recognize that adaptability is an essential component of effective caregiving.

- *Consistent self-assessment and reflection.*

Caregivers should conduct regular self-assessment and reflection. Taking stock of one's physical and emotional health enables proactive identification of stressors and the implementation of coping strategies. Self-awareness is an effective tool for resilience.

### ▪ *Establishing a Strong Support Network*

A strong support system is a lifeline for caregivers. Building relationships with family, friends, and support groups provides emotional support, a forum for sharing experiences, and encouragement during difficult times.

### ▪ *Use Respite Care Services*

Respite care provides caregivers with a temporary break to recharge and attend to personal needs. Whether through professional services or the assistance of family and friends, incorporating respite care into the caregiving plan is critical for avoiding burnout.

### ▪ *Promoting Flexibility and Adaptability*

Dementia caregiving is a dynamic process that necessitates flexibility and adaptability. Caregivers should approach each day with an open mind, embrace change, and adjust strategies to meet the individual's changing needs.

- *Continuous learning and education.*

Staying up to date on dementia and caregiving best practices is an ongoing process. To get the most up-to-date information and strategies, caregivers should seek out educational resources, attend workshops, and maintain contact with healthcare professionals.

- *Celebrating moments of joy and connection*

Despite the difficulties, caregivers should actively seek out and celebrate moments of joy and connection. Recognizing positive moments, whether through shared laughter, meaningful interaction, or a small accomplishment, helps to make caregiving more fulfilling.

■ *Developing Emotional Resilience*

Cultivating emotional resilience is an essential part of managing the caregiving journey. To navigate the emotional complexities of caregiving, caregivers should develop coping strategies, engage in enjoyable activities, and seek professional help as needed.

## Bringing Practical Magic into Everyday Care

■ *Customizing Strategies to Meet Individual Needs*

Dementia care is highly personalised. Caregivers should tailor practical strategies to the individual with dementia's unique needs, preferences, and abilities. Tailoring approaches improve effectiveness and encourage a person-centred care model.

### *Regular communication with healthcare professionals.*

It is critical to maintain open lines of communication with healthcare providers. Regular check-ins enable caregivers to discuss any changes in the individual's condition, seek advice on specific challenges, and ensure that the care plan is in line with changing needs.

### *Collaboration With the Support Network*

The support network is critical to the implementation of practical magic. Collaborating with family, friends, and professionals ensures a unified and comprehensive approach to caregiving, which helps to distribute responsibilities and improves the overall experience.

### ▪ *Understanding the Art of Adaptation*

The art of practical magic is all about adaptation. Caregivers should embrace the fluid nature of caregiving, adjusting strategies in response to feedback, learning from experiences, and incorporating new approaches to improve the effectiveness of daily care.

### ▪ *Recognizing the impact of practical magic.*

Recognizing the power of practical magic is critical for caregivers. Regular recognition of positive outcomes, no matter how minor, reinforces the efficacy of implemented strategies and motivates caregivers to continue their dedicated efforts.

Practical magic weaves compassion, adaptability, and resourcefulness into the intricate tapestry of dementia caregiving. Caregivers who incorporate these practical tips and tricks into daily care can navigate the journey with greater confidence, making each day more manageable and meaningful for both themselves and the people they care for.

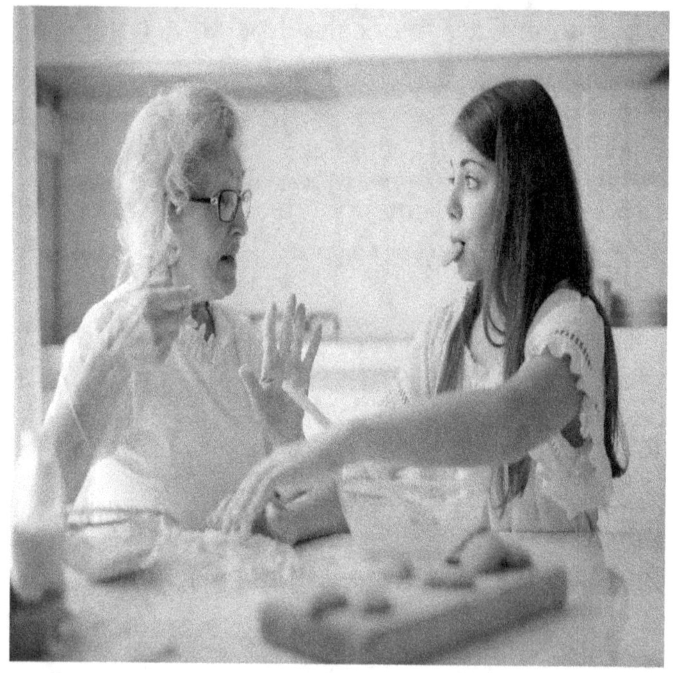

# Chapter 7

# Navigating the Seas of Dementia Care: Strategies for Addressing Challenging Behaviours

Caregivers encounter unique obstacles while caring for dementia patients, especially when confronted with unpleasant conditions and behaviours. In this chapter, we will look at helpful ways for dealing with difficult behaviours connected with dementia. Caregivers will get insights and advice on negotiating difficult situations, resulting in a more peaceful and helpful caring environment.

# *Understanding Difficult Behaviours in Dementia.*

- *Behavioral Changes and Communication*

Individuals with dementia often communicate via challenging actions. As cognitive capacities deteriorate, people may struggle to convey their demands, resulting in dissatisfaction, anxiety, or anger. Understanding these actions as forms of communication is the first step toward successful intervention.

- *Typical Challenging Behaviours*

Aggression, anger, roaming, verbal outbursts, and refusal to care are all examples of challenging behaviours. Identifying the particular behaviour and its triggers is critical for developing targeted measures to address the core causes.

- *Environmental Triggers*

The environment has a tremendous impact in eliciting difficult actions. Loud sounds, strange locations, and crowded areas may all cause tension and discomfort. Identifying and addressing environmental triggers is critical to establishing a more tranquil environment.

## Strategies for Managing Difficult Behaviours

- *Be calm and patient.*

When confronted with problematic behaviours, it is critical to remain calm and patient. Individuals with dementia may mimic the emotions of those around them, therefore a calm and patient demeanour is required to de-escalate situations.

- *Identify and address triggers.*

Caregivers should keep an eye out for and identify the causes of problematic behaviours. Understanding triggers, whether they be particular activities, noises, or times of day, enables proactive intervention and preventative tactics to be implemented.

- *Redirect attention*

Redirecting attention is an effective approach to divert attention away from the problematic behaviour. Introducing a new activity, providing a favourite food, or following a familiar pattern might help to shift attention and relieve stress.

- *Apply Positive Reinforcement.*

Positive reinforcement entails noticing and rewarding desirable actions. When a person demonstrates good behaviour, offering praise, a smile, or a modest reward encourages those acts, resulting in a more happy overall environment.

■ *Develop a Structured Routine.*

Creating a defined routine gives consistency and a feeling of security. Consistent meal times, activities, and rest periods may decrease confusion and anxiety, resulting in a more stable atmosphere.

■ *Offer choices.*

Providing options empowers dementia patients and decreases frustration. Instead of prescribing tasks, caregivers might provide alternatives, giving the client a feeling of control and autonomy.

■ *Ensure Physical Comfort.*

Discomfort, whether caused by pain, hunger, or the need to use the restroom, may lead to difficult behaviour. Physical comfort should be checked on a regular basis, and any pain should be addressed as soon as possible, to avoid and manage difficult circumstances.

- *Use Validation Therapy.*

Validation therapy entails accepting and affirming the individual's emotions and experiences, even if they are not consistent with reality. This strategy promotes trust and rapport while decreasing resistance and problematic behaviours.

- *Seek professional help.*

Healthcare experts, such as dementia specialists, psychologists, or behavioural therapists, may be needed to address challenging behaviours. Seeking expert help enables a thorough grasp of the underlying issues and targeted solutions.

# *Strategies for Commonly Challenged Behaviours*

- *Aggression*

Identifying triggers and putting preventative measures in place are necessary when dealing with aggressive behaviours. Maintaining a safe distance, using soothing language, and adopting diversionary strategies may all assist to de-escalate a crisis.

- *Wandering*

Wandering is a frequent behaviour in dementia. Creating a secure atmosphere, installing door alarms, and offering interesting activities may all assist to divert the individual's attention and lessen the probability of straying.

- *Verbal Outburst*

Frustration or communication challenges might lead to verbal outbursts. Empathy, calm and soothing language, and assistance may all help to diffuse difficult situations.

■ *Care Resistance*

Resistance to care, such as bathing and clothing, may be difficult. Explaining each stage, enabling the person to participate, and adding familiar rituals may all help to make the procedure more pleasant.

■ *Sundown*

Sundowning is defined as increasing agitation and bewilderment in the late afternoon or evening. Creating a peaceful pre-bedtime routine, altering lighting to lessen shadows, and limiting stimulating activities in the evening may all assist control sundowning.

# The significance of regular communication and collaboration

■ *Communication with Healthcare Professionals*

Open contact with healthcare experts is essential. Regular check-ins enable caregivers to address troublesome behaviours, seek intervention advice, and alter care plans to meet the individual's changing needs.

■ *Collaboration with Support Network.*

Collaboration with the support network, which includes family, friends, and professional caregivers, improves the overall effort to manage troublesome behaviours. Sharing experiences, thoughts, and methods creates empathy and support.

■ *Educating and training caregivers*

Caregivers are better equipped to deal with difficult circumstances thanks to education and training. Workshops, seminars, and online resources give useful information on dementia care, behavioural management, and communication tactics.

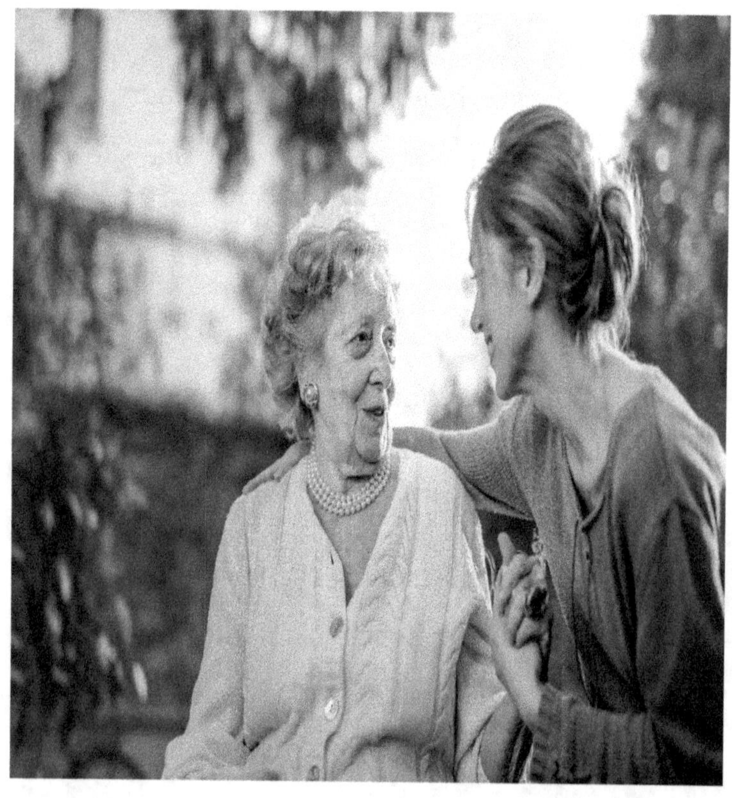

# Chapter 8

# Nurturing the Caregivers: A Guide to Ensuring Personal Wellbeing

Caring for a loved one with dementia is a noble and difficult task that demands unwavering devotion. However, while caring for others, caregivers must prioritise their own well-being. In this section, we will look at caregiver self-care techniques as well as ways for striking a good balance between personal and caring obligations.

## *The importance of personal well-being for caregivers*

- *Understanding the Caregivers' Journey.*

The function of a caregiver in dementia care is diverse. It entails not just satisfying the basic demands of the dementia patient, but also managing the emotional complications that ensue. Recognizing the significance of personal well-being is essential for maintaining the caregiver's physical and emotional health during this rigorous journey.

### ▪ *The Effect of Caregiving on Personal Wellbeing*

Caregiving, although pleasant, may have a negative impact on a caregiver's physical and mental health. The ongoing demands, unanticipated obstacles, and emotional intensity of dementia care need a proactive approach to personal well-being.

## *Self-Care Techniques for Caregivers*

- *Prioritising physical health*

Physical well-being is the foundation of quality caring. Caregivers should emphasise frequent exercise, a well-balanced diet, and appropriate sleep. These core routines help to maintain energy levels, increase resilience, and improve overall physical health.

- *Incorporating relaxation techniques*

Caregivers must prioritise stress management. Incorporating relaxation methods, such as deep breathing exercises, meditation, or mindfulness, reduces stress, boosts emotional well-being, and improves capacity to deal with difficult circumstances.

- *Developing Healthy Sleep Patterns*

Quality sleep is critical for cognitive performance and emotional well-being. Caregivers should develop good sleep habits, provide a sleep-friendly atmosphere, and seek help if sleep difficulties occur. Quality rest has a direct influence on the capacity to deliver effective care.

### ▪ *Promoting Social Connections*

Caregivers often struggle with isolation. Cultivating social relationships, whether via frequent contacts with friends, joining support groups, or participating in community activities, is an important outlet for sharing experiences and getting emotional support.

### ▪ *Participating in Hobbies and Personal Interests*

Personal well-being depends on maintaining a feeling of individual identity. Caregivers should schedule time for hobbies and personal interests, such as reading, doing creative activities, or participating in sports. These activities help to create a more meaningful and balanced lifestyle.

- *Establishing realistic boundaries.*

It is critical to establish clear boundaries between caring tasks and personal time. To prevent burnout and maintain a good work-life balance, caregivers should be aware of their own limits, express their requirements, and establish reasonable goals.

- *Regular Health Checkups*

Monitoring one's own health is sometimes overlooked in favour of caring for others. Regular health check-ups, screenings, and consultations with healthcare specialists help caregivers prioritise their own health and treat any emergent health issues as soon as possible.

- *Seeking Professional Help.*

Caregivers should not hesitate to seek expert assistance when necessary. Therapists, counsellors, and support groups may offer a secure environment for caregivers to express themselves, get help, and learn effective coping skills.

## *Balancing personal life and caregiving responsibilities*

- *Establishing realistic schedules*

Balancing personal life and caring requires thoughtful preparation. Caregivers should make realistic calendars that include personal interests, social events, and time for leisure in addition to caring tasks.

- *Delegating Responsibility*

Caregivers do not have to shoulder the full load alone. Delegating chores to family members, friends, or professional help helps caregivers to split the workload, offering much-needed breaks and promoting a more sustainable caring regimen.

### ▪ *Connecting with Family and Friends*

Open communication with family and friends is critical to achieving a good balance. Caregivers should communicate their requirements, discuss their caring schedule, and request help as needed. A supportive community may provide understanding and aid.

### ▪ *Use Respite Care Services*

Respite care services provide caregivers short pauses to attend to personal needs or just refresh. Whether via professional services or the assistance of friends and family, adding respite care into the caregiving plan is critical for avoiding burnout.

### ▪ *Promoting flexibility and adaptability*

Balancing personal and caring responsibilities necessitates some degree of flexibility. Caregivers should be willing to change schedules, explore alternate solutions, and revise plans in response to the person with dementia's developing demands and their own changing circumstances.

- *Celebrating personal accomplishments.*

Acknowledging personal accomplishments, no matter how minor, is an important part of preserving balance. Caregivers should appreciate times of self-care, personal successes, and the tenacity shown throughout the caring journey.

- *Putting aside quality time for oneself*

Quality time for oneself is a need, not a luxury. Caregivers should set aside time for self-reflection, relaxation, and enjoyable hobbies. These times help to maintain emotional well-being and avoid the degradation of personal interests.

- *Regular evaluation of personal boundaries*

Personal limits change with time, and caregivers should review and adapt them on a regular basis. Recognizing when modifications are required, conveying changes, and maintaining a good balance between caring and personal life is a continuous effort.

## Integrating Self-Care into Daily Caregiving.

- *Integrating Self-Care into Daily Routines*

Self-care should not be an afterthought, but rather an essential component of the daily routine. Caregivers may add minor self-care routines into their caring routine, such as taking brief pauses, reflecting, or participating in a favourite activity.

**■ *Educating the Support Network on Caregivers' Needs.***

Caregivers should actively convey their self-care requirements to their support group. It is critical to educate family and friends on the value of personal well-being and to seek their help in establishing an atmosphere favourable to self-care.

**■ *Review personal goals on a regular basis.***

Setting personal objectives, whether for self-care or individual activities, serves as a road map for sustaining personal well-being. Caregivers should assess and change their objectives on a regular basis to account for changing conditions and priorities.

**■ *Prioritising Self-Care During Stressful Times***

The necessity of self-care is heightened at especially difficult times in caring. Caregivers should emphasise self-care measures, seek extra help, and be proactive in addressing their own needs during times of high stress.

- *Recognizing the Value of Self-Care.*

Recognizing the intrinsic significance of self-care is a fundamental paradigm shift for caregivers. Understanding that personal well-being is not a luxury but a need for successful caring leads to a more sustainable and rewarding caregiving experience.

The thread of personal well-being is carefully woven into the tapestry of dementia caring, altering the whole fabric of the caregiver's experience. Caregivers may traverse the complicated environment with resilience by prioritising self-care, establishing boundaries, and balancing personal and caring duties. This fosters a happier and more sustainable caregiving experience.

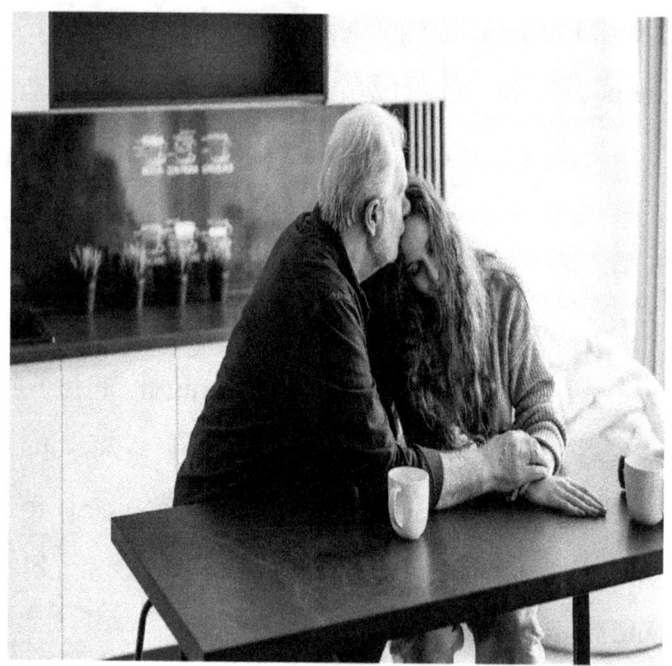

# Chapter 9

# *Crafting Moments of Joy: Engaging Dementia Patients in Meaningful Activities.*

Caring for someone with dementia is a journey that goes beyond the issues of memory loss and cognitive decline. Despite the complexity, generating gratifying moments via meaningful activities has become a cornerstone of dementia care. In this investigation, we will look at several approaches to involve people with dementia in activities that offer them delight and foster relationships via shared experiences.

# *Understanding the significance of fulfilling moments*

**• *The Impact of Meaningful Activities.***

Engaging people with dementia in meaningful activities goes beyond entertainment; it improves their entire well-being. Meaningful activities may elicit good feelings, improve cognitive performance, and foster a sense of purpose and success.

**• *Developing Connections Through Shared Experiences***

Shared experiences create a special link between dementia patients and their caretakers. Creating moments of delight via shared activities develops a relationship that overcomes the barriers of cognitive decline, improving the quality of life for both the person and the caregiver.

# Ways to Engage People with Dementia in Meaningful Activities

- *Adapting Activities to Individual Interests*

Understanding and implementing a person's interests into activities is critical. Whether it's a prior activity, beloved music, or particular areas of interest, adapting activities to personal tastes makes for a more meaningful and pleasurable experience.

- *Sensory Stimulation Activities.*

Sensory stimulation exercises use numerous senses, resulting in a rich and immersive experience. Simple activities such as touching textured textiles, listening to relaxing music, or indulging in fragrant candles may elicit happy feelings and increase cognitive engagement.

- *Interactive storytelling.*

Storytelling is an effective strategy for engaging with people who have dementia. Crafting simple and accessible tales, reminiscing about common events, or using visual aids may elicit memories, promote discussion, and foster a feeling of connection.

- *Artistic expression and creativity.*

Artistic pursuits enable people with dementia to express themselves. Painting, painting, making, and other creative activities allow for self-expression while also instilling a feeling of success and delight.

- *Music and Movement Therapy.*

Music has a unique ability to elicit emotions and awaken memories. Incorporating music and movement into activities, such as dancing or playing popular melodies, not only makes them more enjoyable, but it also increases cognitive and physical engagement.

- *Outdoor Activities and Nature Connection.* Spending time outside and engaging with nature has therapeutic effects. Simple hobbies such as gardening, bird watching, or taking a trip in a local park provide sensory stimulation, fresh air, and a change of scenery.

- *Memory games and cognitive exercises.* Memory games and cognitive activities promote brain function. Puzzles, memory cards, and basic cognitive exercises customised to an individual's ability all help to improve mental agility and well-being.

- *Cooking and baking together.* Cooking or baking with dementia patients leverages on old rituals and sensory experiences. Simple recipes and chores may be tailored to their skills, giving them a feeling of purpose and the satisfaction of producing something together.

## *Creating a Connection Through Shared Experiences*

### ▪ *Creating a Calm and Supportive Environment.*

Creating a suitable atmosphere is critical to effective engagement. A peaceful and friendly environment, devoid of interruptions, fosters a feeling of security, making people with dementia more open to sharing activities.

### ▪ *Active participation and collaboration.*

Encourage active engagement and cooperation to promote a feeling of inclusion. Whether it's working on an art project together, solving a puzzle together, or engaging in a common activity, actively incorporating people with dementia improves the bonding experience.

- *Patience & Flexibility*

Patience is a virtue in dementia care. Individuals may take longer to finish activities or communicate with themselves. Being patient and adaptable, tailoring activities to their speed and interests, guarantees a pleasant and stress-free experience.

- *Nonverbal Communication and Gestures.*

Nonverbal communication, such as gestures and facial expressions, is important for connecting with others. Individuals with dementia may find comfort and understanding in nonverbal signs, enhancing the emotional connection during shared activities.

- *Celebrating Small Achievements*

Recognizing and praising little accomplishments throughout activities fosters a good and supportive atmosphere. Whether it's solving a puzzle, painting a picture, or just enjoying a shared time, recognizing these accomplishments adds to the enjoyment of the event.

▪ *Developing a Routine for Shared Activities*

Establishing a schedule of common activities adds structure and predictability. Consistency in involving persons with dementia in meaningful activities, whether daily or weekly, helps to establish a feeling of regularity and familiarity.

▪ *Keeping a positive attitude.*

Positive attitudes are infectious. Caregivers who maintain a cheerful attitude throughout shared activities contribute to a more uplifting experience. Individuals with dementia often react to the energy and passion of others around them.

**▪ *Capturing and reflecting on shared moments***
Documenting shared events in pictures, notebooks, or scrapbooks provides a concrete record of shared experiences. Reflecting on these times promotes a feeling of connection and serves as a visual reminder of the delight that comes from engaging in meaningful activities.

## *Integrating Meaningful Activities into Daily Care.*

**▪ *Integrating Activities into the Daily Routine***
Meaningful activities must be effortlessly interwoven into the everyday routine. Whether it's beginning the day with a favourite song,

taking a creative break in the afternoon, or closing down with a relaxing sensory exercise, including these moments into the routine makes them more impactful.

**• *Communication with Healthcare Professionals*.**

Maintaining open contact with healthcare experts is critical. Caregivers should share experiences on effective engagement, seek advice on new activities, and discuss any necessary changes depending on the individual's cognitive skills and preferences.

**• *Collaboration with the Support Network*.**

Collaborating with a support network, which includes family members, friends, and professional caregivers, improves the efficacy of group activities. Sharing ideas, experiences, and resources promotes a wide and stimulating variety of activities.

- ***Customizing Activities Based on Progress and Preferences.***

Individuals with dementia may have changes in their preferences and talents over time. Caregivers should constantly tailor activities to these changes, ensuring that the engagement stays relevant and pleasurable.

- ***Regular assessments and adjustments***

Regularly analysing the effect of activities on the well-being of dementia patients enables caregivers to make educated decisions. Monitoring replies, recording preferences, and soliciting feedback all contribute to the continuous improvement of the engagement approach.

In the fabric of dementia care, meaningful activities and shared experiences weave bright patterns of pleasure and connection. Caregivers may create a narrative of satisfaction for themselves and people they care for by adapting activities to specific interests, creating a peaceful atmosphere, and actively engaging in shared experiences.

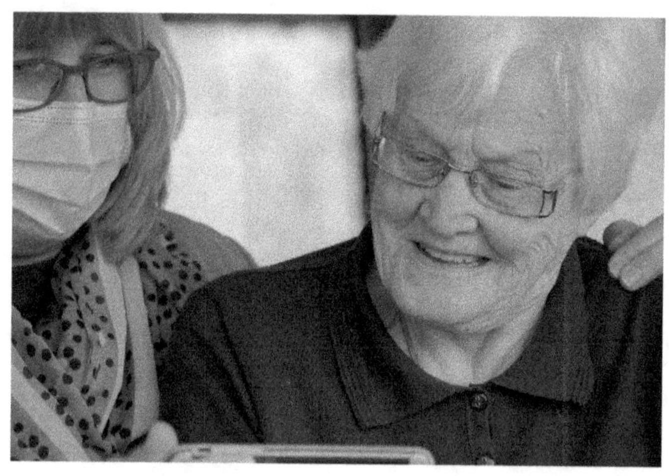

# Chapter 10

# Navigating Care: When to Seek Professional Help and Access Support Services for Caregivers

Caring for someone with dementia is a huge and difficult duty that requires steadfast devotion. Recognizing when to seek professional assistance and obtaining support services are critical components of safeguarding the well-being of both the person with dementia and the caregiver. In this study, we will look at the indicators that signal a need for professional help, the many sorts of healthcare experts engaged in dementia care, and the range of support services accessible to caregivers.

# _Recognizing the Signs: When To Seek Professional Help_

- **_Behavioral and cognitive changes._**

Obvious changes in behaviour and cognition, such as greater confusion, memory loss, or personality abnormalities, may indicate the need for professional help. Healthcare specialists that specialise in dementia may do examinations to evaluate the level and kind of cognitive loss.

- **_Safety concerns_**

If the safety of the person with dementia or others is jeopardised due to wandering, aggressiveness, or difficulty with everyday routines, professional assistance is required. Occupational therapists and safety specialists can help you create a secure atmosphere.

- **_Reduction in Physical Health_**

Dementia often presents physical health concerns. Healthcare specialists such as physiotherapists or home health aides may be required if mobility declines, medicines are difficult to manage, or personal hygiene is neglected.

### *Uncontrollable Emotional Stress for the Caregiver*

Caregivers face a significant emotional toll, and when stress gets excessive, finding help is critical. Mental health specialists, such as psychologists or counsellors, may provide caregivers emotional support and coping skills.

### *Difficulties in Daily Care.*

As the responsibilities of daily care grow increasingly complicated, caregivers may find it helpful to speak with experts. Occupational therapists, nurses, and social workers may provide practical guidance on how to manage everyday chores and improve care.

- *A lack of social engagement.*

Isolation is a major problem for people with dementia and their caretakers. Social workers and support organisations may help caregivers connect with others experiencing similar issues, forming a helpful network.

## Healthcare professionals caring for dementia

- *Neurologists and Geriatricians.*

Neurologists and geriatricians are experts in the diagnosis and treatment of neurological disorders, including dementia. They are responsible for performing examinations, giving prescriptions, and providing general medical advice.

## ■ *Psychiaters and Psychologists*

Mental health professionals, such as psychiatrists and psychologists, provide assistance to both the person with dementia and their caregiver. They can help with behavioural and emotional difficulties by providing therapy and coping strategies.

## ■ Occupational Therapists.

Occupational therapists work to improve a person's ability to perform daily activities. They can offer practical solutions for managing daily routines, enhancing safety, and preserving independence for as long as possible.

## ■ *Speech and Language Therapists.*

Speech and language therapists help people with dementia who have trouble communicating. They can offer strategies for improving communication and addressing speech and language issues.

### ▪ *Physiotherapists*

Physiotherapists focus on physical rehabilitation. Physiotherapy for dementia patients can help with mobility issues, muscle strength maintenance exercises, and overall physical well-being.

### ▪ *Home health aides*

Home health aides provide practical assistance with daily tasks, personal care, and health monitoring. Their assistance enables people with dementia to remain in familiar surroundings while receiving necessary care.

### ▪ *Social workers*

Social workers play an important role in connecting caregivers with resources and support services. They can help with navigating healthcare systems, obtaining financial assistance, and offering emotional support.

- *Hospice and palliative care specialists*

Hospice and palliative care specialists can provide compassionate end-of-life care to people with advanced dementia. They prioritise comfort, symptom management, and support for both the patient and their family.

## *Accessing Caregiver Support Services*

- *Support Groups*

Joining caregiver support groups provides an invaluable opportunity to share experiences, receive emotional support, and gain insights into coping with the challenges of dementia care. These groups can be both local and online, giving caregivers more options.

## ▪ *Respite Care Services*

Respite care services provide caregivers short pauses to attend to personal needs or just refresh. Whether via professional services or the assistance of friends and family, adding respite care into the caregiving plan is critical for avoiding burnout.

## ▪ *Educational workshops and training*

Educational workshops and training sessions provide caregivers with the knowledge and skills required for effective dementia care. These sessions cover communication strategies, behavioural management, and self-care.

## ▪ *Financial assistance programs*

Managing the financial aspects of dementia care can be difficult. Social workers can help caregivers get access to financial assistance programs, grants, and benefits that help them cope with the financial burden of caregiving.

### ▪ *Adult Daycare Services*

Adult day care services offer a structured and supervised environment for people with dementia, giving caregivers time for work or personal activities. These programs provide social and cognitive stimulation.

### ▪ *Home Modification Service*

As dementia progresses, changes to the home may be required for safety and access. Home modification services can advise on adaptations such as handrails, ramps, and other safety measures.

### ▪ *Legal and planning assistance.*

Legal and planning assistance assists caregivers with legal issues such as establishing power of attorney or creating advanced care directives. Seeking professional advice in these areas ensures that the legal aspects of caregiving are adequately addressed.

- *Telehealth Services*

Telehealth services enable remote access to healthcare professionals and support services. This convenient option enables caregivers to seek advice, attend consultations, and obtain information without the need for in-person visits.

## *Navigating the Healthcare System:*

- *Developing a Comprehensive Care Plan*

Caregivers can collaborate with healthcare professionals to create a comprehensive care plan that addresses the individual's dementia-specific needs. This plan describes the medical, emotional, and practical aspects of care.

- ***Maintain Regular Communication with Healthcare Providers.***

Maintaining open and regular communication with healthcare providers is critical. Caregivers should share updates on the individual's condition, report any changes, and seek advice on how to handle specific challenges.

- ***Advocate for the Individual's Needs***

Caregivers advocate for the people in their care. Advocating for the individual's needs ensures personalised and compassionate care, whether during medical consultations, care planning meetings, or interactions with support services.

- ***Staying Aware of Treatment Options***

Understanding available treatment options, such as medications and therapies, enables caregivers to make informed decisions. Keeping up with the latest developments in dementia care improves the quality of care provided.

- *Seeking a Second Opinion*

Obtaining second opinions in complex medical situations can provide new perspectives and insights. It ensures that caregivers have a thorough understanding of the patient's condition and available treatments.

## Chapter 11

# Navigating the Maze: Financial and Legal Considerations for Dementia Care

Caring for a loved one with dementia is a journey that includes not just emotional and physical difficulties, but also complex financial and legal issues. Understanding the difficulties of navigating the financial environment and dealing with legal issues is critical to ensure the well-being of both the dementia patient and the caregiver. In this examination, we will look at the financial and legal sides of dementia caring, providing insights into future planning and developing a complete framework that protects the interests of all parties involved.

# _Unravelling the Financial Tapestry._

- ### _The Costs of Dementia Care_

Caring for a person with dementia has financial ramifications. Caregivers must be aware of the possible expenditures connected with dementia care, which include medical fees and specialised care services. Medication, medical visits, in-home care, assisted living facilities, and, in certain situations, memory care units are examples of these expenses.

- ### _Insurance coverage_

Understanding the coverage offered by health insurance is essential. Different insurance plans may provide varied amounts of coverage for dementia-related expenditures. Medication, treatments, and, in certain cases, long-term care are all covered. Caregivers should evaluate plans, question about coverage details, and look for extra insurance choices if necessary.

- *Financial planning and budgeting.*

Financial planning is an essential part of dementia care. Caregivers may efficiently control expenditures by creating a thorough budget that takes into account both current and prospective future spending. This might include talking to a financial counsellor about investment possibilities, assessing retirement funds, and developing long-term financial stability initiatives.

- *Investigate Government Assistance Programs*

Government-sponsored aid programs may be quite beneficial. Individuals with dementia may qualify for financial help via programs such as Medicaid, Supplemental Security Income (SSI), and Veterans Affairs benefits. Accessing these critical resources requires successfully navigating the qualifying requirements and application procedures.

 *Legal Considerations in Financial Planning.* Integrating legal issues into financial planning is critical for preserving the interests of the person with dementia and their family. Creating powers of attorney, trusts, and guardianship alternatives are all legal choices that may give clarity and guarantee financial problems are handled correctly.

## Legal Framework: Protecting Rights and Interests

### ▪ *Power of Attorney*

Granting power of attorney enables a person to choose someone to make financial and legal choices for them. This legal document is an effective tool for managing a person with dementia's financial affairs. Caregivers should ensure that powers of attorney are created while the person is still competent to make appropriate choices.

## ▪ *Living wills and advanced directives*

A living will and advance directives define a person's intentions for medical care if they become unable to communicate. Addressing concerns like life-sustaining measures and end-of-life care ensures that medical choices are consistent with the individual's beliefs and desires.

## ▪ *Guardianship.*

If a person with dementia is no longer able to make choices and has not appointed a power of attorney, guardianship may be required. Guardianship is a legal procedure in which a guardian is appointed by a court to make decisions on behalf of an incapable person.

## ▪ *Establishing Trust*

Trusts are legal instruments that enable assets to be administered on behalf of a person with dementia. Establishing trusts may give an organised approach to managing financial matters, ensuring that assets are utilised for the individual's advantage and that a chosen trustee administers them wisely.

- *Assessing Legal Capacity*

Assessing an individual's legal capacity is critical in establishing their ability to make financial and legal choices. Seeking expert counsel from lawyers or healthcare specialists may help you understand when and how legal ability exams should be undertaken.

## *Planning for the Future*

- *Long-term care planning.*

Long-term care planning is a proactive step that includes thinking about whether you could require assisted living, nursing home care, or specialist dementia care. Long-term care insurance, if available, may be a helpful tool for paying the expenses of these services.

*Estate planning*

Estate planning is arranging and structuring one's assets to ensure they are transferred in accordance with the individual's preferences. This involves creating wills, identifying beneficiaries, and dealing with tax issues. Consulting with an estate planning attorney ensures that the legal framework is consistent with the individual's objectives.

- *Reviewing and updating legal documents*

Because dementia advancement may impair decision-making skills, legal papers must be reviewed and updated on a regular basis. This contains powers of attorney, living wills, trusts, and other pertinent paperwork. Regular assessments guarantee that legal frameworks are accurate reflections of the individual's current desires and circumstances.

- ***Consulting with legal and financial professionals.***

Engaging with legal and financial specialists is an essential component of future planning. Attorneys that specialises in elder law, financial consultants, and estate planners may offer personalised counsel, address particular issues, and walk caretakers through the complexities of legal and financial preparation.

- ***Communication and Documentation.***

Effective family communication is critical when preparing for the future. Transparent talks regarding financial and legal problems, the individual's preferences, and future obstacles help to build a common understanding. Documenting these talks and conclusions in paper promotes clarity and serves as a helpful reference in the future.

## *Interplay between Financial and Legal Considerations*

■ *Coordination among financial and legal professionals*

Collaboration among financial and legal specialists is required for comprehensive dementia care planning. To ensure that all sides of the caring journey are in sync, lawyers, financial advisers, and other relevant experts must communicate openly.

■ *Educating Caregivers in Financial and Legal Matters*

Empowering caregivers with financial and legal understanding is a proactive strategy. Educational programs, tools, and consultations may provide caregivers with the knowledge they need to make sound choices and negotiate the difficulties of dementia care.

- *Monitoring and adjusting financial plans.*

Dementia is a degenerative disorder, therefore financial strategies must be flexible to suit changing circumstances. Regular monitoring and revisions to financial plans, taking into account changing care requirements and prospective changes in income or costs, ensure that the financial framework stays solid.

- *Legal Protections against Financial Exploitation*

Dementia patients are particularly susceptible to financial abuse. Implementing legal measures, such as restricting access to bank accounts or appointing a trusted representative, may assist protect against exploitation or financial abuse.

### ▪ *Think about charitable giving and philanthropy.*

For families with the resources and desire, including charity, giving into their financial plans may be a rewarding experience. Consulting with financial advisors may assist people in exploring choices for supporting organisations they care about while maintaining a long-term financial strategy.

# Chapter 12

## Strengthening Bonds: Using Community Resources and Joining Caregiver Support Groups.

Caring for someone with dementia is a difficult journey that demands both fortitude and a network of support. In addition to providing care at home, caregivers may benefit greatly by accessing community services and participating in caregiver support groups. This dual approach promotes a feeling of belonging, gives extra help, and assures that caregivers are not facing the problems of dementia care alone.

# _Community Resources: A Supportive Pillar_

- **_Community Aging and Disability Services_**

Caregivers benefit greatly from local ageing and disability programs. These programs often include information, counselling, and assistance customised to the specific needs of older persons and those with disabilities, including those with dementia. Connecting with these agencies may provide access to a range of community-based help.

- **_Community Health Clinics & Outreach Programs_**

Community health clinics and outreach organisations often host dementia-related events, seminars, and educational sessions. Caregivers may get access to critical information, learn new caring skills, and network with specialists who can provide direction and help.

- ***Adult Day Care Centers.***

Adult day care centres are community-based organisations that provide organised services to older persons, including those with dementia. These centres provide caregivers with respite while ensuring that people with dementia participate in meaningful activities in a secure and supervised setting.

- ***Senior centres and recreational programs.***

Senior centres and leisure programs commonly provide events for older persons. Caregivers may look into these programs to provide their loved ones with dementia chances for socialising, mental stimulation, and physical exercise, therefore improving their overall well-being.

- *Faith-based organisations and community groups.*

Prayer groups, counselling services, and community outreach are common ways for faith-based organisations and community groups to help caregivers. These networks may provide emotional and spiritual support, fostering a feeling of community that extends beyond the practical requirements of caring.

- *Transport Services*

Transportation may be a huge difficulty for caregivers and dementia patients. Many cities provide transportation services particularly for older folks, ensuring that they can attend medical appointments, community activities, and social events.

- *Legal Assistance and Advocacy Services*

Legal assistance and advocacy services are critical in assisting caregivers with navigating legal issues relating to dementia care. These services may help with concerns including guardianship, powers of attorney, and obtaining government assistance.

- *Meal Service and Food Delivery Programs*

It is critical to ensure that patients with dementia have enough nourishment. Community-based meal services and food delivery programs may offer healthy meals, easing the load on caregivers and ensuring that their loved ones are fed.

## *Joining Caregivers' Support Groups: A Network of Understanding*

- *Online Caregiver Forums*

The digital era has made it easier to set up online caregiver forums and support groups. Caregivers may use these platforms to share their stories, get advice, and connect with others who are experiencing similar issues. Online forums have the benefit of accessibility and a wide variety of opinions.

■ *Local In-person Support Groups*

Local in-person caregiver support groups encourage face-to-face connection and develop a feeling of community. These groups are often organised by healthcare facilities, community centres, or non-profit organisations, and they allow caregivers to exchange experiences and learn from others in their area.

■ *Specialized Support Groups for Dementia*

Dementia-specific support groups are designed to address the special issues that caregivers of dementia patients experience. These groups often include guest speakers, instructional workshops, and a forum for discussing dementia-specific topics, resulting in a supportive atmosphere customised to the needs of caregivers in similar circumstances.

### ▪ *Phone Helplines and Hotlines*

Telephone helplines and hotlines provide rapid access to expert advice and emotional assistance. Caregivers may use these programs for urgent guidance on issues like dealing with difficult behaviours or finding resources during a crisis.

### ▪ *Therapeutic support groups*

Therapeutic support groups, led by experienced therapists or counsellors, explore the emotional elements of caring. These meetings provide a secure area for caregivers to express themselves, manage stress, and build coping methods for the emotional issues that come with dementia care.

### ▪ *Residential Caregivers' Communities*

Residential caregiver communities bring together those who are caring for loved ones with dementia. These communities provide a shared living environment, resulting in a built-in support network for caregivers to share tasks, experiences, and provide mutual aid.

- ***Education Workshops and Seminars***

Educational workshops and seminars allow caregivers to improve their knowledge and abilities. These seminars often include subjects such as effective communication tactics, stress management, and understanding the evolution of dementia, providing caregivers with the knowledge they need to provide optimal care.

- ***Counseling and Therapy Services***

Counselling and therapy services may help caregivers maintain their mental health. Professional counsellors may provide individual or group therapy sessions to help caregivers deal with the emotional effect of caring and learn coping methods.

## *Maximising the benefits: A Dual Approach.*

- *Balancing Community Resources and Support Groups.*

The most successful way to dementia care is to strike a balance between using community services and joining caregiver support groups. Community resources give practical aid, whilst support groups provide emotional and social support, resulting in a full network of care.

- *Tailoring Support to Individual Needs*

Caregivers should customise their interactions with community services and support groups to meet the specific needs of their loved ones and themselves. Customising the support network ensures that caregivers get help that is tailored to the individual issues they confront throughout their caring journey.

- *Regular check-ins and updates.*

Staying connected to community resources and support groups requires frequent check-ins and updates. Caregivers should be proactive in searching out new possibilities, attending events, and staying in touch to ensure they are getting the most out of the resources available.

- *Advocating for Increased Community Support*

Caregivers play an important role in pushing for more community assistance. Caregivers may help enhance and expand services for people in similar circumstances by actively engaging in community initiatives, offering input, and sharing their experiences.

- *Embracing the Strength of Shared Experience*

Participating in caregiver support groups strengthens the value of shared experiences. Caregivers in these groups often take peace in knowing that they are not alone in their problems, which fosters a feeling of camaraderie and understanding that may be deeply soothing.

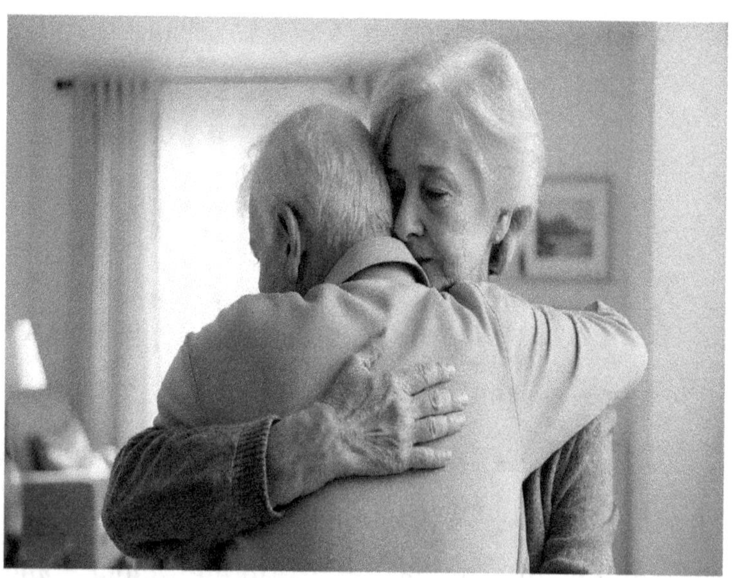

# Chapter 13

# Nurturing Bonds: The Importance of Staying Connected in the Caregiving Journey

Caring for a loved one with dementia is a serious and sometimes difficult job that may lead to feelings of loneliness. Caregivers and their loved ones must maintain social and emotional connections in order to thrive. In this investigation, we will look at the importance of maintaining social ties and ways for overcoming the isolation that often accompany the caring journey.

# *The Value of Maintaining Social Connections*

- ***Emotional Support and Understanding***

Staying in touch with friends, family, and a larger social circle offers emotional support and understanding. Caregivers who share their stories with others find comfort in knowing they are not alone in their struggles. Emotional connections become an important source of strength while managing the complications of dementia caring.

- ***Decreased Stress and Anxiety***

Social relationships provide a buffer against the stress and worry that often accompany caring. A support network enables caregivers to share the load, get help when required, and find moments of rest. The mere act of discussing problems and getting supportive replies may dramatically reduce stress.

■ *Preventing Caregiver Burnout.*

Isolation may contribute to caregiver burnout. Caregivers who remain connected may share duties, take breaks as needed, and avoid the crushing tiredness that can come with the constant demands of dementia care. Social ties prevent mental and physical exhaustion.

■ *Establishing a sense of normalcy.*

Maintaining social relationships gives caregivers a feeling of normality in their life. Participating in discussions, activities, and shared experiences outside of caring helps caregivers keep their identity and interests. This balance promotes a healthy emotional state.

■ *Improving Mental Well-being*

Isolation is a proven risk factor for the development or worsening of mental health problems. Regular social connections, whether in person or digitally, promote mental well-being. Conversations, laughing, and shared moments of delight all contribute to the caregiver's positive attitude and view on life.

- *Developing a Supportive Ecosystem*

Social relationships offer a supportive environment for caregivers. Friends and family members who understand the difficulties of dementia caring may give practical advice, share information, and lend a listening ear. This environment serves as a source of strength for caregivers during challenging times.

# *Combating Isolation on the Caregiving Journey*

- *Prioritising Social Activities.*

Caregivers should include social activities as part of their daily routine. This might involve frequent trips, social meetings, or participation in community activities. Caregivers actively battle the propensity to retreat into solitude by putting social ties first.

- *Utilising Technology for Virtual Connections*

In the present day, technology provides an effective tool for remaining connected. Caregivers may communicate with friends and family via video calls, social media, and messaging applications, regardless of geographical distance. Virtual connections provide flexibility and convenience.

- *Participating in caregiver support groups.*

Caregiver support groups provide a dual role by offering both emotional support and useful knowledge. Joining these organisations, whether in person or online, allows caregivers to interact with people who understand their situation. It offers a platform to share experiences, seek advice, and establish a network of support.

- *Seeking Respite Care Services.*

Respite care services allow caregivers to take a break and participate in social activities without worrying about their loved one's health. Respite care, whether via professional services or support from friends and family, allows caregivers to spend crucial time socialising.

- *Discovering Community Events and Activities*

Participating in community events and activities broadens social circles. Caregivers might look into area events, interest clubs, and volunteer opportunities. Participating in these activities not only strengthens relationships, but also gives caregivers a feeling of purpose outside of their caring job.

- *Communicating openly with loved ones.*

Open communication with loved ones is crucial. Caregivers should convey their desire for social ties and explain how friends and family members might help them retain such relationships. Clear communication ensures that the caregiver's social needs are known and honoured.

- *Schedule regular outings.*

Integrating frequent trips into the caregiving routine is critical. Whether it's a stroll in the park, a coffee date with friends, or attending cultural events, these activities provide caregivers a change of scenery and opportunity for social engagement.

- *Integrating Social Time into Daily Care.* Caregivers might include social time in their everyday care tasks. For example, allowing friends or family members to participate in activities with the person with dementia not only strengthens social relationships but also fosters delight and shared experiences.

# Conclusion

## Embracing Resilience in the Dementia Caregiving Journey

As we approach the end of our search for knowledge of the complex terrain of dementia care, it becomes clear that this journey is both a struggle and a tremendous opportunity for development. The essential topics underlined emphasise the significance of a comprehensive strategy that includes compassion and empathy for all areas of care.

Staying connected emerges as an essential component for caregivers, offering emotional support, lowering stress, and minimising burnout. The importance of maintaining social relationships cannot be stressed as caregivers face the specific challenges of dementia.

Our excursion delved into the importance of community resources and the important assistance they provide. From local ageing services to adult day care facilities, these options provide a safety net for caregivers, offering practical aid as well as a feeling of community.

Joining caregiver support groups stands out as a strong way to develop understanding and unity. In these meetings, caregivers share their experiences, learn new things, and develop friendships that reinforce their determination. The shared journey serves as a source of motivation, reminding caregivers that they are not alone in facing hardships.

Achieving a delicate balance between financial and legal factors is an important part of future planning. Caregivers may safeguard their loved ones' well-being and traverse the complexity of the caring environment with confidence if they grasp the complexities of these issues and seek expert assistance.

Soothing approaches, inspirational coping suggestions, and practical magic create a tapestry of solutions to improve the caring experience. Caregivers are armed with strategies that assist not just people in their care, but also their own well-being, such as establishing quiet settings and having a good outlook.

Finally, caregivers are urged to see their position as a journey full of chances for connection, development, and resilience. The obstacles may be daunting, but the benefits of giving compassionate care to a loved one with dementia are tremendous. As caregivers continue along this journey, may they find strength in the relationships they have made, consolation in shared experiences, and a great feeling of satisfaction in the important effect they make every day.